How to Reduce the Chances of a Heart Attack

by M. Usman

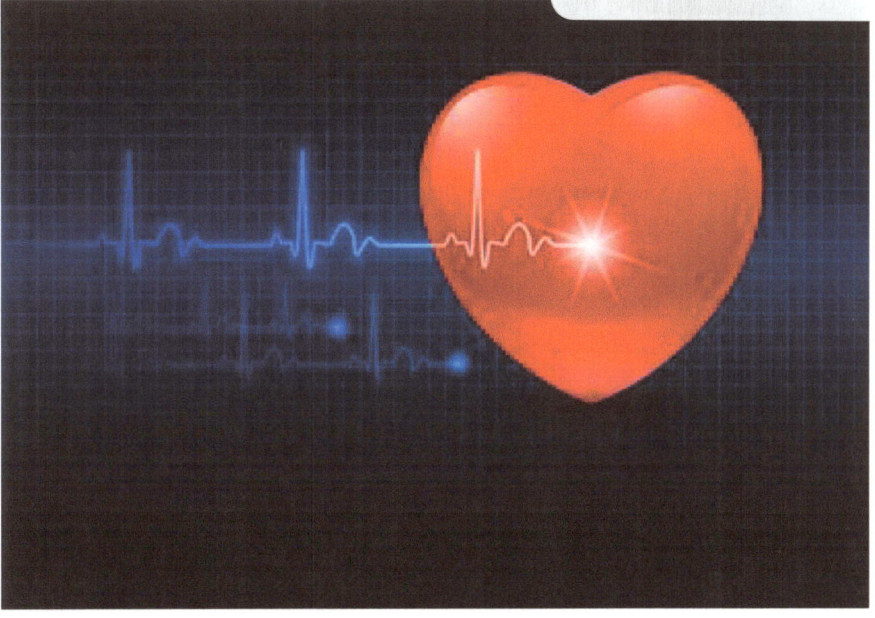

Health Learning Series

Mendon Cottage Books

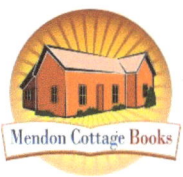

JD-Biz Publishing

Disclaimer

The information is this book is provided for informational purposes only. It is not intended to be used and medical advice or a substitute for proper medical treatment by a qualified health care provider. The information is believed to be accurate as presented based on research by the author.

The contents have not been evaluated by the U.S. Food and Drug Administration or any other Government or Health Organization and the contents in this book are not to be used to treat cure or prevent disease.

The author or publisher are not responsible for the use or safety of any diet, procedure or treatment mentioned in this book. The author or publisher is not responsible for errors or omissions that may exist.

Warning

The Book is for informational purposes only and before taking on any diet, treatment or medical procedure it is recommended to consult with your primary care provider.

Our books are available at

1. Amazon.com
2. Barnes and Noble
3. Itunes
4. Kobo
5. Smashwords
6. Google Play Books

Table of Contents

Introduction

Imagine that you are breezing through life and life seems to be going so smoothly ; you are so full of life that you do not even have the time to look after yourself, much less others. Visit to your doctor can wait, of course, because right now nothing is wrong with you. You are perfectly okay. And then one day you are running to congratulate your son, who has perhaps just graduated from his high school or maybe you are getting late for some appointment and suddenly, an excruciating pain arises in your chest and goes to your shoulder... you want it to subside but the pain keeps gripping you. You feel as if your life is at an end. But you don't want it to end. There is so much to do. But you can't stand on your feet anymore. You feel yourself falling, falling, falling and may be you won't wake up again.

The above account describes heart attack in a nutshell. And according the American Heart Association,

"About 7, 25,000 Americans have a heart attack each year"

So, it's quite common, common enough that someday I and you could encounter this situation too. However, it's not like we can't do anything about it. While there's no vaccine for heart attack, we can, however, significantly reduce the chances of getting a heart attack by making simple changes in our routines. This book will attempt to highlight the fact that you can, by knowing about heart attack and what risks it poses, make subtle changes in your routine and diet that will go a long way towards reducing the risk of heart attack. I must emphasize here, however, that this is no reference book and it can reinforce but cannot replace a good doctor's advice. So, while I assure you that you will find it very informative and helpful, do not rely solely on this book for curing a heart attack; instead consult a doctor as well. With this caution in mind, let us now first see what this heart attack, which takes away the lives of so many people each year, really is, before diving into what we can do to avoid it.

SECTION 1: HEART ATTACK – AN OVERVIEW

Chapter 1: Heart Attack – a crumbling of your heart

Part 1 – Defining heart attack

Heart! Such an amazing organ in the chest, pumping blood throughout the whole body around 72 times a minute. Just as an engine runs a car, the heart is responsible for running a human. And so when this engine of the human body falters, it has drastic consequences for the body. This, in a nutshell, is a heart attack.

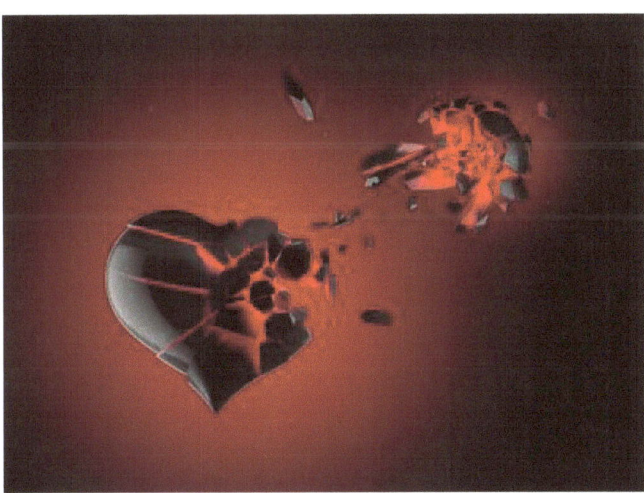

The heart muscle, owing to its continuous activity, needs a continuous supply of oxygen and nutrients to keep pumping the blood. So, any condition which cuts off blood supply and, as a result, the supply of oxygen and nutrients to the heart muscle, the heart muscle suffers greatly. Initially function of heart cells is depressed which is followed by permanent death of the cells if the blood supply is not restored quickly. This is associated with severe pain in the chest and a variety of other symptoms which we'll get to in a later chapter. All these symptoms together constitute a heart attack. So, now we can attempt a definition of the condition that is known as heart attack.

'A heart attack is the death of, or damage to, part of heart muscle because the blood supply to the heart muscle is severely reduced or stopped'

So, just as an engine requires fuels for its successful operation, heart requires blood. And when this fuel is compromised heart attack is the result.

Part 2 - Causes of a heart attack

Now the question arises: "What causes this cut off of the blood supply to the heart?"

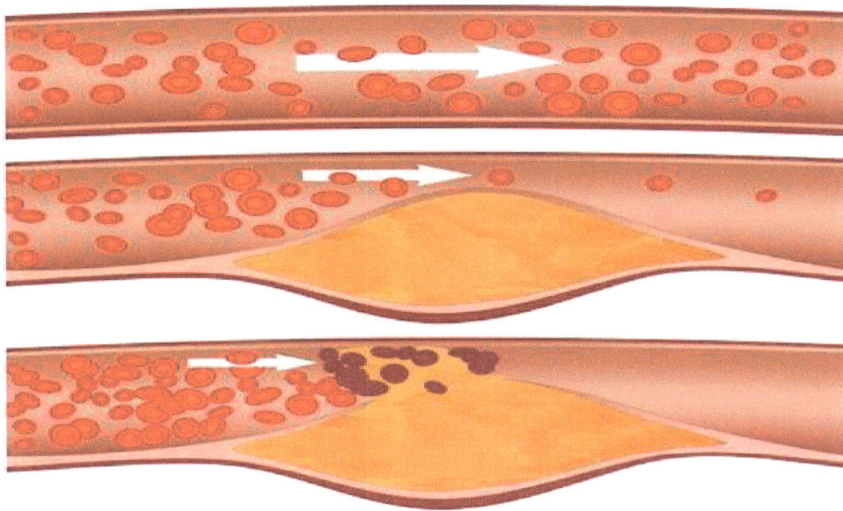

The answer to this is that the heart is supplied blood by a large number of blood vessels which are called coronary arteries (Latin – cor = heart). These arteries are responsible for maintaining the supply of oxygen and nutrients to the heart muscle. Consider these vessels to be like pipes of a car which provide fuel to the engine. If I, for some reason, obstruct fuel in one of these pipes, naturally the performance of the engine will suffer. If I obstruct most of the pipes, the engine, getting no new fuel and having consumed all the residual fuel, will stop altogether. Such a condition occurs in the heart during a heart attack. This "obstruction of the pipes" occurs primarily due to one of the following causes:

- **Coronary heart disease:** Heart attacks most often occur due to coronary heart disease. This disease is characterized by the narrowing of the lumen of the vessels due to the deposition of wax-like plaques called atherosclerotic plaques in the walls of the vessels. The plaque then narrows down the lumen of the vessel and eventually obstructs it completely so that the blood can no longer flow through the vessel and this cuts off the blood supply to the heart muscle supplied by that vessel. This appears to be the most important cause of heart attack in the majority of the patients. What causes the formation of these plaques, you ask? It's actually the fats in our blood (especially cholesterol) which deposit in the vessels throughout our lives and this deposition becomes a problem especially in the old age. An unhealthy life style is the major reasons of this diseases. Lack of proper and regular exercise; eating junk food increases the quantity of harmful cholesterol in our blood. This cholesterol, in turn, causes coronary artery disease.

- **Clot formation in coronary arteries:** A clot arising locally or from the peripheral circulation may lodge in the small coronary arteries; eventually it may obstruct the whole lumen and cause complete blockage of blood flow through the artery.

- **Spasm of coronary arteries:** Sometimes, a coronary artery may undergo spasm (tightening). This will result in reduction and may be even complete stoppage of flow through the artery. This is a rare cause. This is mostly present in association with an atherosclerotic plaque. However, spasm may even occur in the absence of atherosclerosis.

It is worth noting here, that in most cases, not one but a combination of these factors is present and they together contribute to the drastic loss of blood supply to the heart muscle, causing a life threatening situation – the heart attack.

Chapter 2: Symptoms – When you know it's coming...

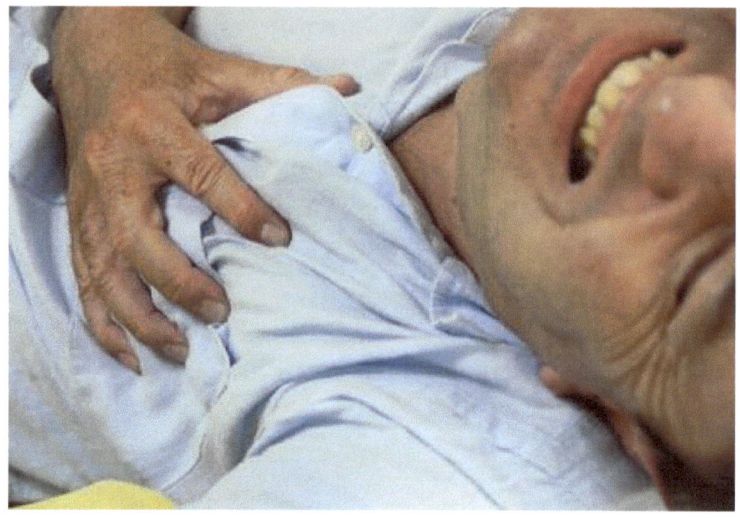

Dark clouds in the sky with lightning and heavy winds signal a thunderstorm and a diligent farmer puts his harvest under a shelter to avoid damage by the storm. So, as nature warns the farmer, does nature warn humans when the thunderstorm of heart attack falls upon them? Well, yes indeed. Kind nature does that too. And if you are diligent enough, you can avoid not only the damage, but you can prevent the thunderstorm altogether. All you need is to know the symptoms which signal a heart attack.

Not all heart attacks begin with excruciating pain in the chest as shown in the movies or TV shows. In one study for example, a third of the patients with heart attack had no chest pain. The main symptoms which are mostly associated with heart attack are as follows:

1. **Chest pain or discomfort:** Chest pain or discomfort is the most common symptom that signals a heart attack. The discomfort

usually begins in the center of the chest or left side of the chest. The discomfort can feel like uncomfortable pressure, squeezing, fullness, or pain. It lasts for a few minutes and may come and go. This is because of the substances that are released from the dying heart muscle which excite the sensory pain nerves.

2. **Upper body pain:** The pain may radiate beyond the chest to shoulder, arm, back, neck, teeth and jaw. This upper body pain may sometimes be present even in the absence of chest discomfort. This is because the sensory nerves supplying these upper parts of the body share common roots with nerve supplying the heart which gives the sensation of pain in the areas supplied by these nerves (i.e. the upper body parts)

3. **Stomach pain:** The pain may extend into the abdomen for the same reason as mentioned for upper body pain.

4. **Shortness of breath:** This is characterized by panting and heavy breathing. This may occur before chest pain and may even be present in the absence of chest pain.

5. **Light headedness:** This is marked by dizziness and feeling that one is about to fall.

6. **Anxiety** and the person feels confused. It becomes difficult for him to make decisions.

7. **Nausea and vomiting.**

Most heart attacks begin with mild symptoms with discomfort preceding severe pain. When such a thing occurs, the important thing is to recognize that it's signaling a very serious condition and not ignore these symptoms. Calling an ambulance in such a situation may be life saving and changing your routine will be necessary to prevent the occurrence of such symptoms again.

Chapter 3: Risk factors – The heart breakers

Why do certain people get heart attacks while others do not? Why do some get it at a relatively younger age while others when they are very old? The answer to this is that there are certain risk factors: heart breakers that break down your heart (literally) and the people who have these heart breakers will, inevitably, get their hearts « broken » by a heart attack at some point of their life.

In order to effectively prevent heart attacks, we must know what predisposes a person to heart attack. The major risk factors which make a person likely to develop heart attack are:

1. **Age:** The older a person gets, the more fat deposits in his/her arteries and the more the chances of heart attacks. Accordingly, males older than 45 years of age and females older than 55 years are more likely to get a heart attack than younger males and females. Aging also weakens the muscles of heart.

2. **Smoking:** Smokers (including people with secondhand smoke exposure) are 2-4 times more prone to develop coronary heart disease (atherosclerosis) as compared to non-smokers. This is because the chemicals which are present in it damage the internal walls of arteries.

3. **High blood cholesterol:** Cholesterol, as mentioned earlier, is the major component of atherosclerotic plaques responsible for heart attacks. Increased blood level of wrong kind of cholesterol (LDL cholesterol) is likely to cause narrowing of arteries.

4. **High blood pressure:** When the blood pressure is high, it damages the walls of arteries and accelerates the formation of plaques and clots which in turn obstruct the arteries causing heart attack.

5. **Diabetes:** A diabetic individual with a high blood glucose level is more prone to develop heart attack.

6. **Obesity:** Obesity is a risk factor because it inevitably leads to uncontrolled blood cholesterol, blood pressure and diabetes. Reducing obesity by just 10 percent can reduce this risk.

7. **Lack of physical activity:** An inactive lifestyle contributes to obesity and high cholesterol levels. So, regular exercise (especially strenuous exercise) is very beneficial for the heart.

8. **Other risk factors** include family history of heart attack, drug usage, stress and history of preeclampsia.

It would be worth noting here, that while we cannot do anything about some of the risk factors such as age, we can willingly reduce many of the risk factors including obesity, high cholesterol and high blood pressure. All that is needed is the will to do so.

Chapter 4: Grave prognosis – why you should bother trying to avoid a heart attack...

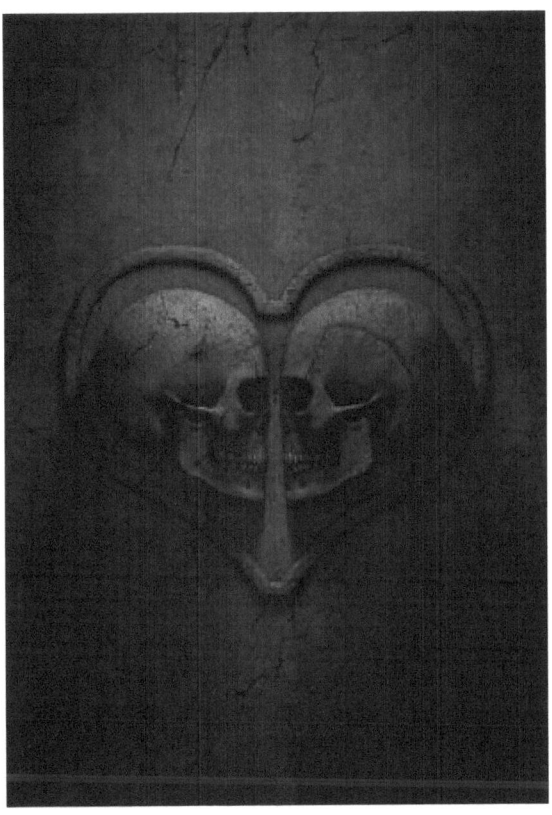

When asked about their heart problems, many a brave patients talk casually about them. What could go wrong? They've been well throughout their lives and they are so sure that the pain they feel is nothing but some indigestion which will go away in a day or two. However, the doctors well know the gravity of the situation and the danger this little "indigestion" can pose. So, the first thing that a person MUST do to avoid heart attack, is realize the gravity himself.

So, let me totally be honest with you: Heart attack is very often fatal. An untreated heart attack will lead to the following:

1. Abnormal heart rhythms (arrhythmias): Damaged heart muscle will lead to abnormal circuits to develop in the heart. So even if the damage is not very severe, the abnormality of rhythm will make the heart an ineffective pump.

2. Heart failure: Untreated heart attack will progress to the point that a large portion of heart muscle becomes non-functional. At this point, the heart will fail to pump enough blood to meet the requirements of the body. This is the condition of heart failure.

3. Heart rupture: Areas of heart muscle damaged by the lack of blood supply can lead to the rupture of that portion of heart.

4. **DEATH:** Arrhythmias, heart failure and heart rupture will often cause death within a few minutes of heart attack unless immediate medical treatment is given.

So, this life, to which we cling to so dearly, will fade away with a heart attack. And while a grave prognosis awaits those who ignore their condition, those who are diligent enough to realize the dangers in time are rewarded with a very healthy prognosis and a longer life span. I'm sure you and I want to be in the latter category.

Section II: Reducing Heart attacks

Chapter 5: Effective prophylaxis – an introduction

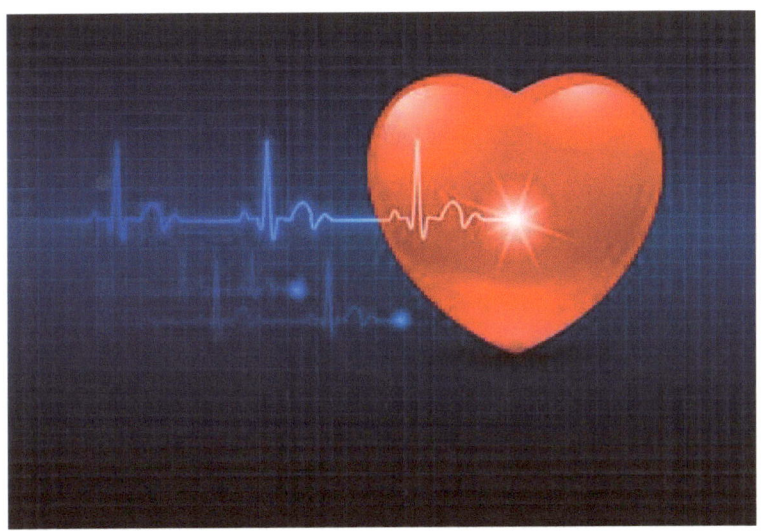

It's better to be safe than sorry. No one wants to die. And I'm sure that any method that will help prevent a life threatening event, will be more than welcomed by every man on the planet. Once a heart attack has occurred or the conditions have aggravated to the point that heart attack is imminent, there is little anyone can do to avoid damage to the heart. Although modern medicine does allows some reduction of the damage, however, it is far better to avoid the heart attack altogether. This prophylaxis is suggested for everyone, especially for people who already have a history of a heart attack.

An effective regimen for heart attack prophylaxis includes non-medication strategies as well as many medicines that'll help you avoid altogether or reduce the conditions that lead to a heart attack. They may be used alone or in conjunction with one another. The latter is more effective of course. Many of these strategies act by improving the blood flow through the coronary arteries which supply the heart muscle. Non-medication strategies do this by preventing the risk factors that lead to the formation of clots and by lowering harmful fat in blood. Medicines act similarly either by reducing the harmful fat or by reducing the clotting of blood. That there is a direct relation between acting upon these prophylactic measures and reduction in the incidence of heart attacks, is a fact that is well established. So, effective prophylaxis is the only defense that we have to avoid a deadly fate of heart attack.

Chapter 6: Non-medication measures – Who needs a doctor ?

Sometimes we do not need to contact professionals. Why bother a carpenter, if all that was needed was to tighten a nail of a chair ? Why would a person go to an electrician if all that was needed to be done was to plug in the wire in the correct socket ? By simply making certain life style changes, we can so effectively prevent a heart attack that there is no need to go to a doctor. These measures can be used alone but when the situation aggravates, medicines are added. However, they together form the first step and the most effective step in reducing heart attacks and without them medicines may not be so effective.

1. **Dietary changes :** Having a diet which is rich in fat and cholesterol and low in fiber increases the risk of heart attack greatly. There are several dietary changes that you can make which will significantly reduce the chances of heart attack.

   - Reduce intake of all Trans and saturated fatty acid. Trans fatty acids are most dangerous. So, you must reduce the amount of foods that contain these fats including red meat, full dairy products, fried foods, packaged foods, margarine and processed baked goods.

   - Increase the intake of fruits and vegetables. Several studies suggest that eating fruits and vegetables especially green vegetables and vitamin C-rich fruits can reduce the chances of heart attacks.

☐ Eat a diet that is rich in vitamins especially vitamin E, folic acid and vitamin B6. All these are anti-oxidants and have been related to reduction in chances of heart disease.

☐ Don't eat too much. Although what you eat is important, how much you eat is also important. Refrain from overeating because that can lead to excess fat, cholesterol and calorie intake.

2. **Say NO to smoking :** Smoking is the leading preventable cause of heart attacks. The chemicals in a cigarette smoke damage the heart and blood vessels. However, the good news is that by quitting smoking you can dramatically reduce the chances of heart attack. Risks of cardiovascular disease begin to decline within months of quitting smoking and reach the levels of persons who have never smoked within 3 to 5 years.

3. **Regular exercise:** Regular exercise can greatly reduce the chances of heart attack. When used in conjunction with other non-medication strategies, the benefit is even greater. Physical activity not only helps to control weight but also helps to avoid other conditions that put a strain on the heart including high cholesterol, diabetes and high blood pressure. In addition strenuous exercise can cause collaterals to develop in the coronary arteries so that if one artery is blocked by a clot, blood flows through alternate paths, thus avoiding a heart attack. So a regular exercise of 30 to 60 minutes will go a long way in preventing a heart attack.

4. **Put a check on your weight:** Obesity is a major risk factor for development of heart attack. Increasing weight will inevitably lead to

high blood cholesterol, high blood pressure and diabetes. So, putting a check on weight is a must. This can be done by controlling the amount of food a person takes in daily and also by regular exercise. Reducing weight will thus significantly reduce the chances of heart attacks.

5. **Stress management:** Excessive stress has been linked to high lipid levels and increased risk of adverse cardiovascular events. Also increased stress is linked to non-compliance of treatment. Relaxation methods, yoga and stress management techniques can all help to reduce the stress.

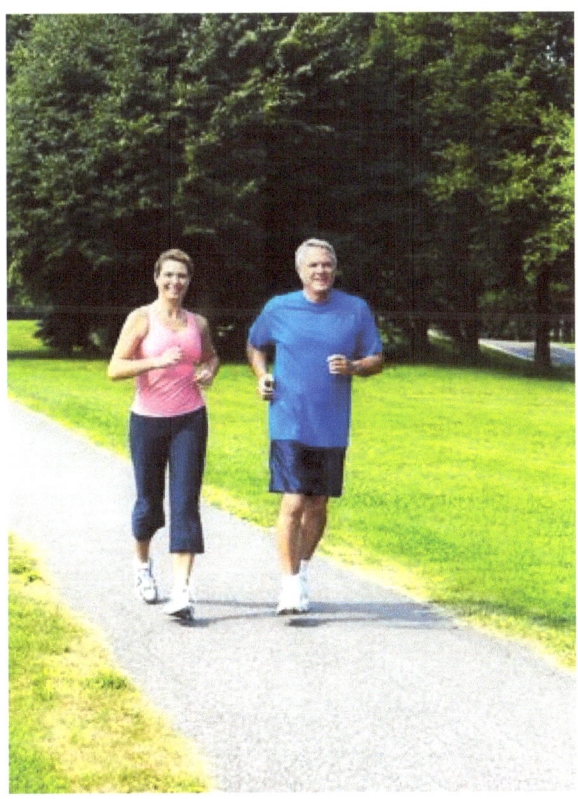

6. **Herbs and nutritional supplements:** The herbs and nutritional supplements which have been found to be useful in reducing the risks of heart attack include the following :

- Turmeric
- Ginger
- Ginkgo
- Garlic
- Onion
- Folic acid
- Vitamin B12
- Vitamin B6
- Bilberry
- Fungreek
- Fish oil
- Magnesium
- Carnitine
- Niacin

So, intake of these nutritional supplements can help to reduce the risks of heart attack significantly.

7. **Get regular checkups:** You must get yourself checked regularly to see what the condition of your body is and whether your non-medication strategy is working well in controlling heart attack or not. Also see a doctor whenever you have any slight suspicion of aggravating heart. This way damage will be prevented before it happens.

It's worth noting here, that for effective prophylaxis, all the above are a must. Even when a person is taking medications these strategies supplant the effect of medications and thus are invaluable to every person who wants to avoid a heart attack.

Chapter 7: Medicines used for prophylaxis – well, sometimes you do (need a doctor)

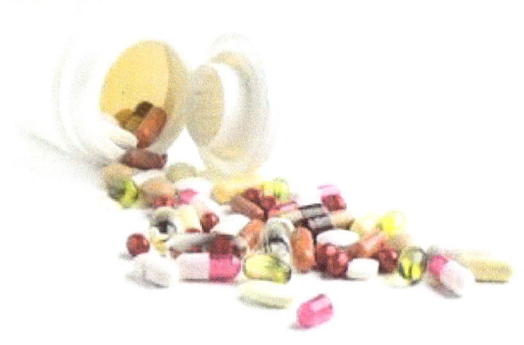

While non-medication strategies are very important, a point may come when they aren't sufficient for controlling the risk of a heart attack. At this point, the only choice left is to use certain medicines which are quite effective in reducing the chances of heart attacks. Also a person with a previous history of heart attack may find that non-medication therapies are insufficient to prevent future attacks. And so like a person, who has tried utmost himself to fix his television and failed and goes to the electrician trusting that the electrician will know better, sometimes non-medication strategies aren't enough and at these times we must consult a doctor instead of trying on stubbornly to cure ourselves without medicines.

Medicines for prophylaxis reduce the heart attacks mostly by reducing blood cholesterol, increasing blood supply to the heart or preventing the formation of clots. Let us now look at these medicines one by one.

1. **Anticoagulants :** These are also known as blood thinners although they do not actually thin the blood. These include heparin, warfarin, tinzaparin and enoxaparin. As mentioned earlier, the primary reason that causes heart attack is a block of coronary arteries. This is due to the formation of a clot. The anticoagulants decrease the clotting ability of the blood so that the chances for formation of new clots are minimized. They don't dissolve existing clots and so cannot be used for the immediate treatment of heart attack but they do prevent the existing clots from getting larger and causing serious problems. So by decreasing the formation of new clots, they decrease the chances of blockage of coronary arteries, supplying the heart muscle and so decrease the chances of heart attack.

2. **Antiplatelet agents :** Antiplatelet agents include aspirin, ticlopidine and dipyramidole. Platelets are small cellular fragments in the blood which help in the clot formation by aggregating together and releasing factors which cause the blood clotting factors to activate. These drugs prevent the platelets from aggregating and thus reduce the formation of clots. When platelet aggregation is suspected these drugs are invaluable in preventing the obstruction of coronary arteries. And so they also reduce the chances of heart attack by reducing clot formation.

3. **Statins :** This class of drugs includes statins, resins and nicotinic acid. These lower the blood cholesterol levels. These have different mechanisms of actions. Some work in the liver, some in the intestine and some reduce the circulation of cholesterol through the blood. However, all have one common result i.e. they all reduce bad quality (LDL) cholesterol and increase the good quality (HDL) cholesterol in the blood. By reducing the « bad » cholesterol levels in the blood, these drugs reduce the formation of atherosclerotic plaques in the coronary arteries and thus reduce the chances of heart attack.

4. **ACE (Angiotensin converting enzyme) inhibitors :** ACE inhibitors include captopril, enalapril, fosinopril and lisinopril. Angiotensin is an endogenous substance that causes the blood vessels to contract and increases the resistance to flow of blood through them. These drugs (ACE inhibitors) inhibit the formation of angiotensin by blocking the enzyme that forms the active form of angiotensin. And so they expand blood vessels and decrease the resistance to blood flow. This leads to an increase in blood flow to the heart muscle and can reduce the load on the heart which in turn prevent heart attack.

5. **Angiotensin receptor blockers (ARBs) :** These drugs include candesartan, losartan and irbesartan. Rather than blocking the enzyme for the formation of angiotensin, these drugs block the receptors on which angiotensin acts and so many of their effects are same as that of angiotensin converting enzyme (ACE) inhibitors except that they are more selective and have fewer adverse effects as compared the ACE inhibitors.

6. **Diuretics :** Commonly used diuretics are chlorthiazide, hydrochlorthiazide, chlorthalidone and furosemide. These drugs increase the elimination of fluid from the body through the kidneys. This reduces the total amount of fluid in the body which in turn reduces the load on the heart. These drugs are also invaluable in reducing the blood pressure which has a further beneficial effect on heart attack prophylaxis.

7. **Beta blockers :** Beta blockers or beta-adrenergic blocking agents include acebutolol, atenolol, betaxolol, bisoprolol, carteolol, metoprolol and nadolol. They decrease the heart rate and cardiac output. The heart beats more slowly and with less force. This leads to a decrease in blood pressure. And so by decreasing the blood pressure, these drugs reduce the formation of atherosclerotic plaques, reducing the chances of heart attacks. Note however that their effectiveness in preventing heart attack has recently been challenged by the Journal of American Medical Association (JAMA).

Although the above medicines can effectively prevent heart attacks, they will be of little use if the risk factors (outlined in Chapter 3 of first section) aren't eliminated by the non-medication prophylactic measures (outlined in Chapter 2 of second section) their usefulness may be offset and heart attack episodes may occur even when a person is regularly taking these drugs. So for effective prophylaxis, both non-medication and medication measures are required. The choice of a particular medication, however, varies with the patient and depends on the presence or absence of other diseases and the other drugs that the patient is taking.

Chapter 8: Work plan – monitor your progress

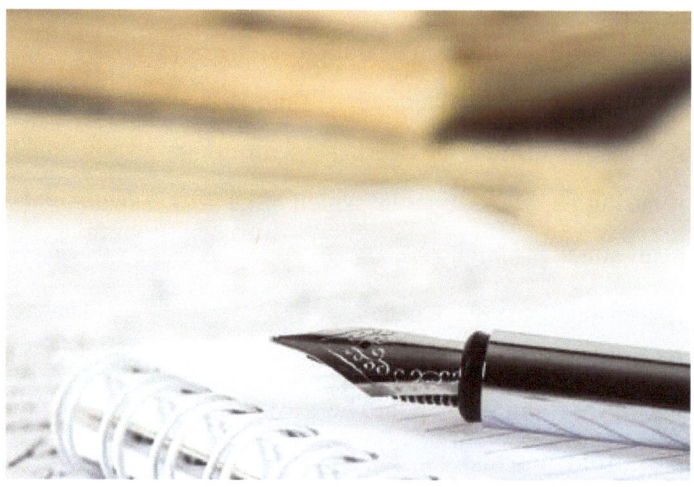

I think it would be fruitless if a person tediously tries to mend his broken bike only to find out after several hours that he has been making no progress in fixing the bike at all. All the hard work would be in vain. So, for good prophylaxis only the measures aren't enough. You must be very wary for even the slightest symptoms of deterioration of your heart and you must monitor your progress continuously to see if the strategy you are following is actually working or not. The advantages of following this strategy are two fold :

1. You'll get more confidence in your prophylactic measures and you will try harder in the future.
2. If the measures aren't working well, then you will know that you must try some other measure.

Following are the main parameters by which you can effectively monitor your progress :

WEIGHT :

1. Carefully monitor your weight : As we age, we get more prone to weight gains because our physical activities decline at an older age. So, you must regularly check your weight. If your weight is increasing, then you should immediately reduce dietary intake and start physical exercises.

2. Calculate your body mass index : To see whether your weight is appropriate for your height or not, the best index is body mass index. A BMI of 25 or higher is considered overweight and associated with increased risks of cardiovascular disease. So, you should regularly monitor your BMI and strive to keep it under 25.

3. Use a tape to measure your waist : A measurement of 40 inches or above is considered overweight for men and a measurement of 35 inches or above is considered overweight for women. Because abdominal fat is especially dangerous and a risk factor in heart disease, measuring waist circumference will help you keep a check on this dangerous parameter. You should immediately do abdominal exercises if you find that your waist circumference is increasing.

BLOOD PRESSURE :

1. **Monitor your blood pressure carefully** : Monitoring blood pressure is essential because higher the blood pressure, the more the chances of formation of atheromas in the coronary arteries. If you find that your blood pressure is excessively high, you must immediately use some medications to reduce the chances of heart attack.

2. **Charting your blood pressure at regular intervals** : The blood pressure measurement that a physician takes at his office is like a

snapshot which doesn't tell him the complete story of what happens throughout the day. So patients are advised to monitor their blood pressure continuously at home and make a chart out of it. This way the physician will get a more complete idea of what is going on inside your vessels.

BLOOD CHOLESTEROL LEVELS:

In the prophylaxis for heart attack, the importance of blood cholesterol has been repeatedly emphasized in this book. So you should regularly monitor blood cholesterol levels to see whether your « bad » (LDL) cholesterol level is going down or not. If it is not going down, then you must use medications in addition to dietary changes.

So, a regularity in prophylactic measures plus regular monitoring of these parameters is necessary for effectively reducing the chances of heart attack.

Chapter 9: Conclusion

Heart attack poses a great challenge to humanity. The number of deaths occurring through heart attacks is staggering. To face this challenge the best method is to use ways and measures to avoid such a condition. So if you want to be safe rather than sorry later, you must take all the measures that are possible. Most of these measures have been highlighted in this book. Use this book in conjunction with the advice of a good doctor. This way, I assure you that you will have significantly increased your life span.

Photo credits

All images licensed by fotolia.com

Seniors couple jogging.

© *Kurhan - Fotolia.com*

Opened notepad, fountain pen and books

© *Becker - Fotolia.com*

Cholesterol plaque in artery (atherosclerosis) illustration

© *Diamond_Images - Fotolia.com*

Abstract Heart Monitor

© *dvarg - Fotolia.com*

medicine bottle

© *Paulista - Fotolia.com*

No Smoking Sign

© *akarb - Fotolia.com*

Gothic valentine

© *grandeduc - Fotolia.com*

hommeinfarctus

© *dalaprod - Fotolia.com*

broken heart

© *sowanna - Fotolia.com*

Author Bio

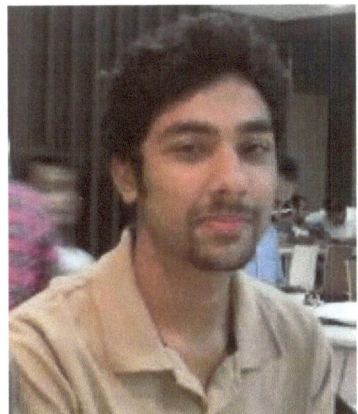

Muhammad Usman is a distinguished medical graduate of Allama iqbal medical college (AIMC). He is a professional writer who has been in the field for more than 4 years. During this time he has produced 10,000+ articles, blogs and eBooks on various niches related to diseases, health, fitness, nutrition and well being. He is a regular contributor to several journals related to medicine and surgery. He is the editor of several journals and newspapers.

Check out some of the other JD-Biz Publishing books

Gardening Series on Amazon

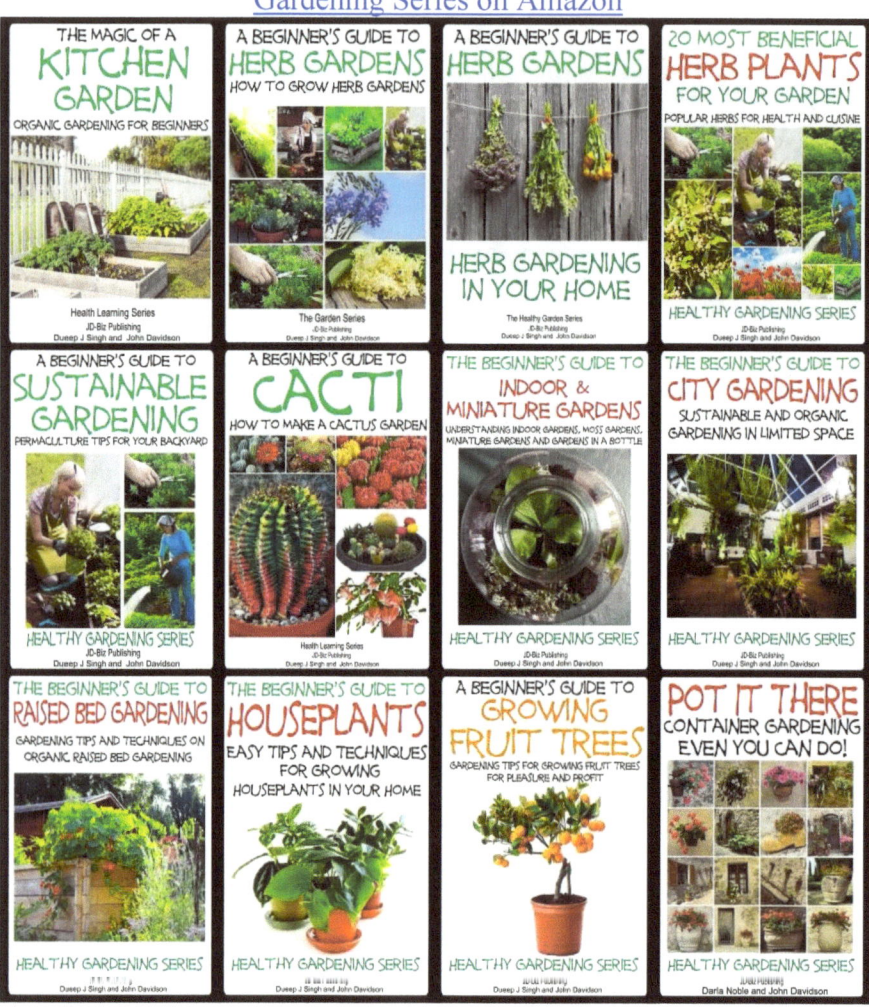

Download Free Books!
http://MendonCottageBooks.com

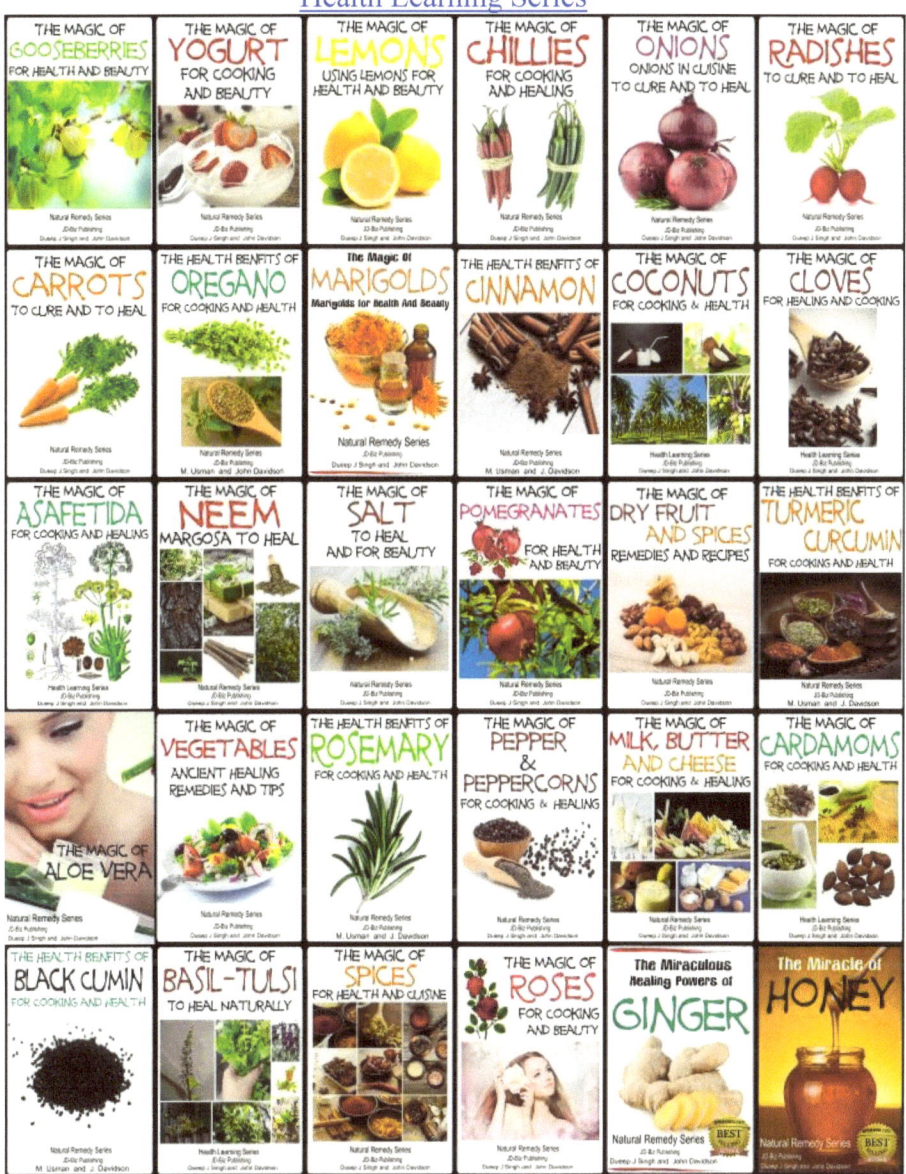

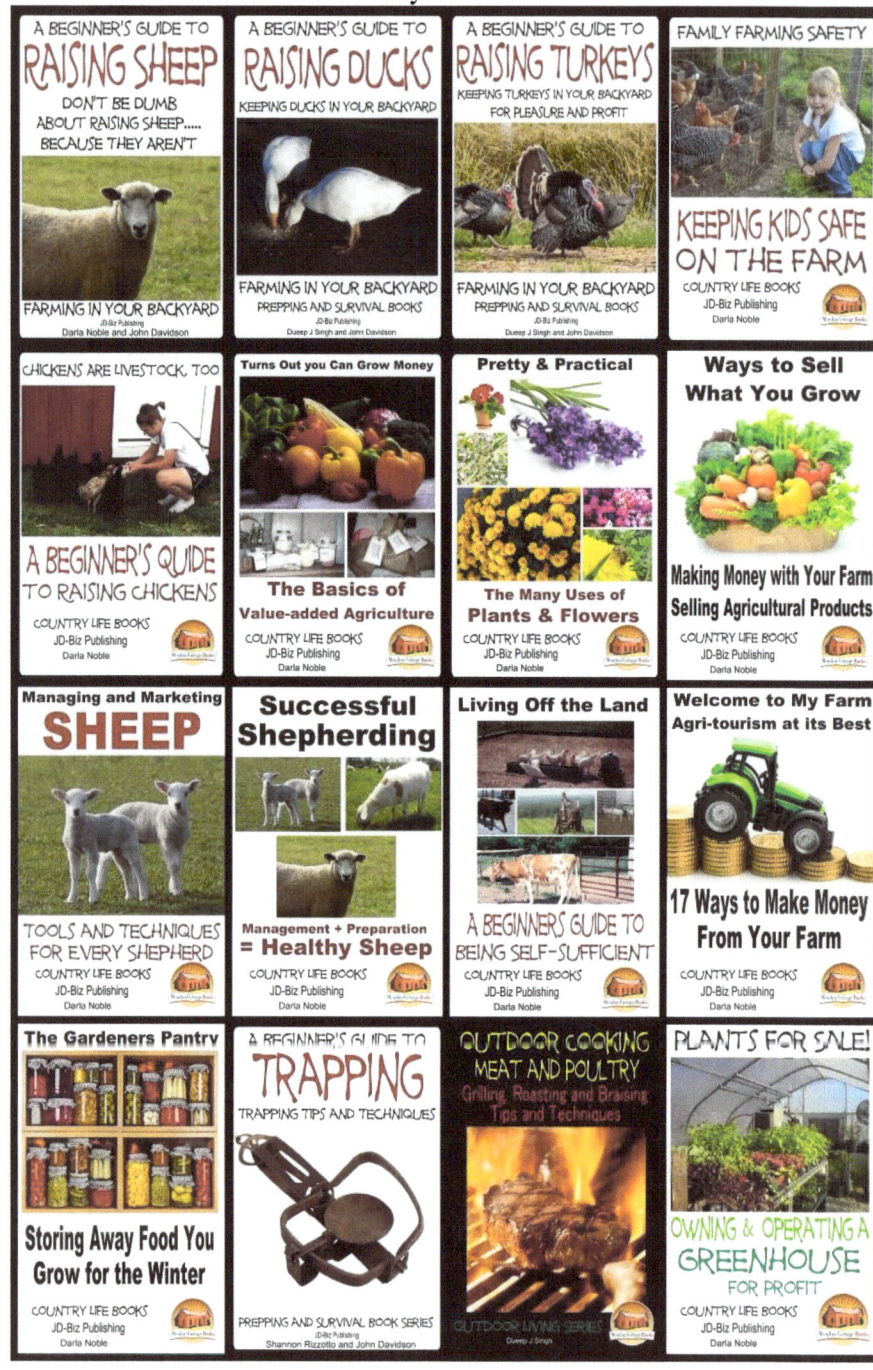

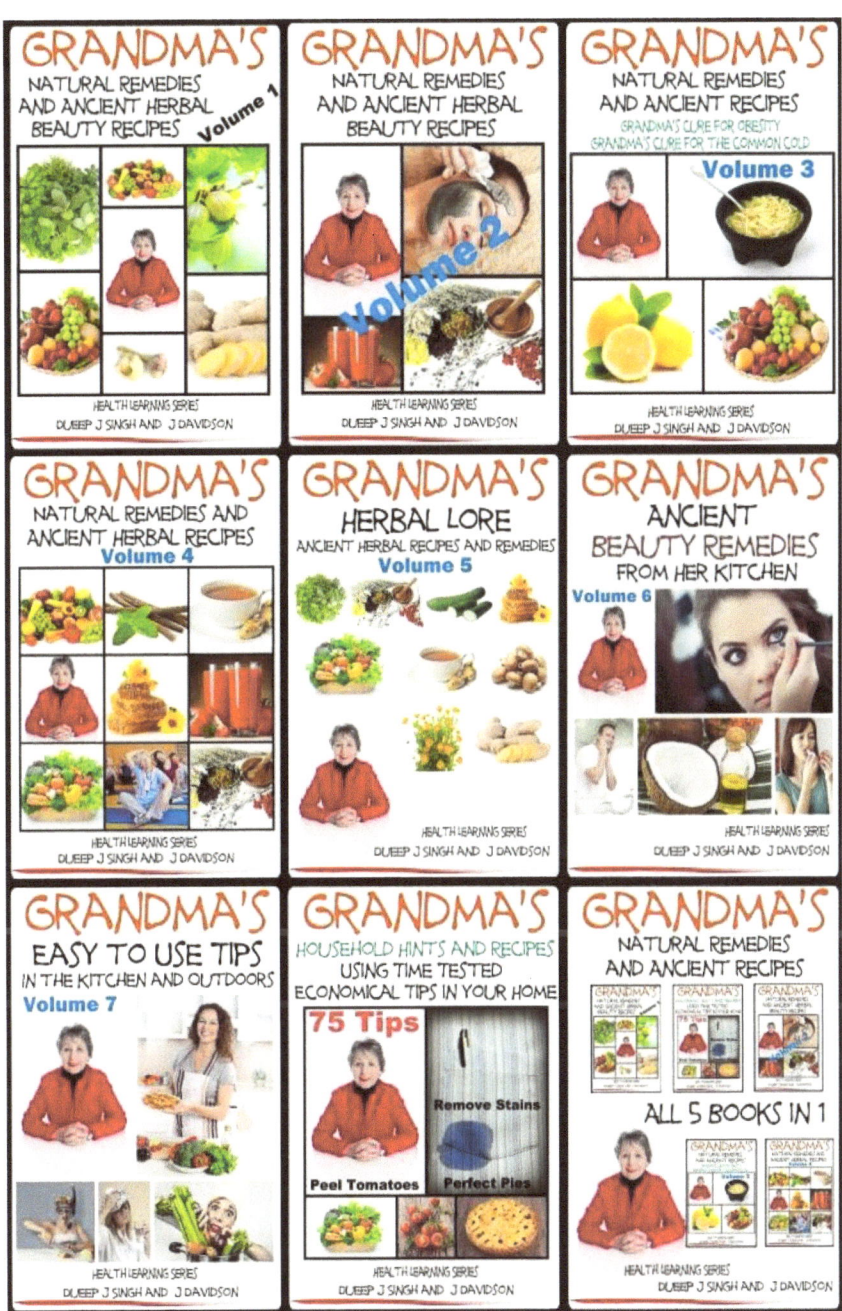

Health Learning Series

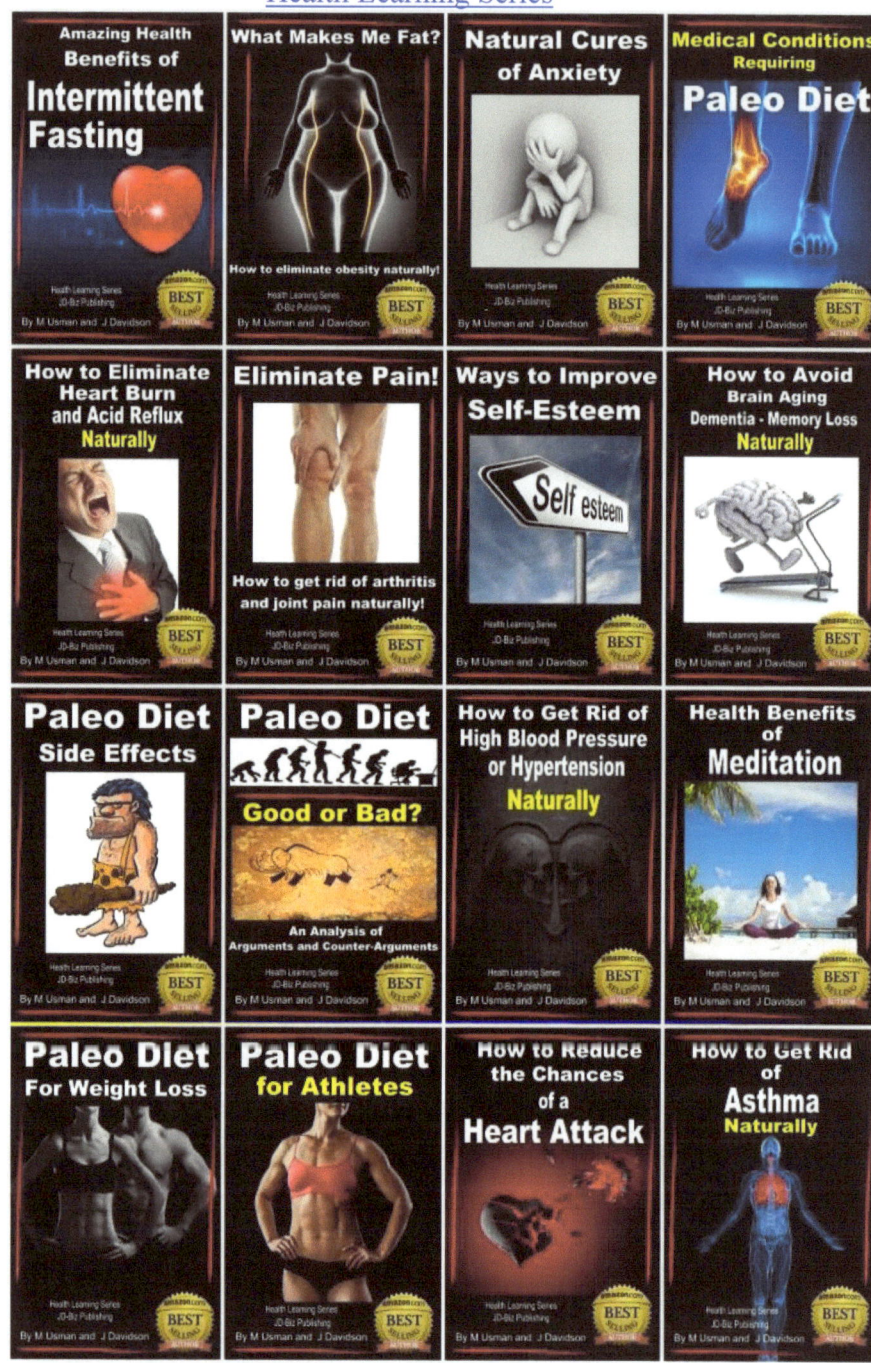

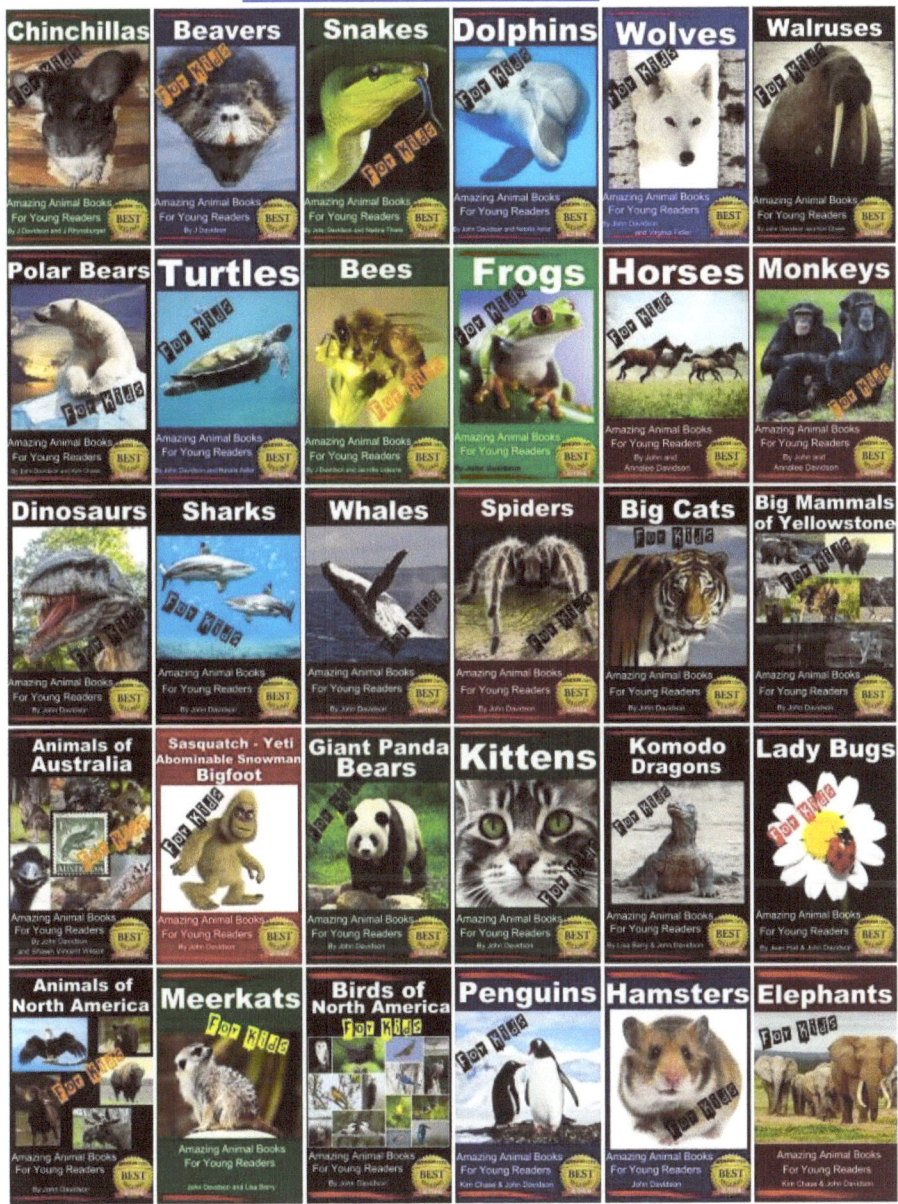

Learn To Draw Series

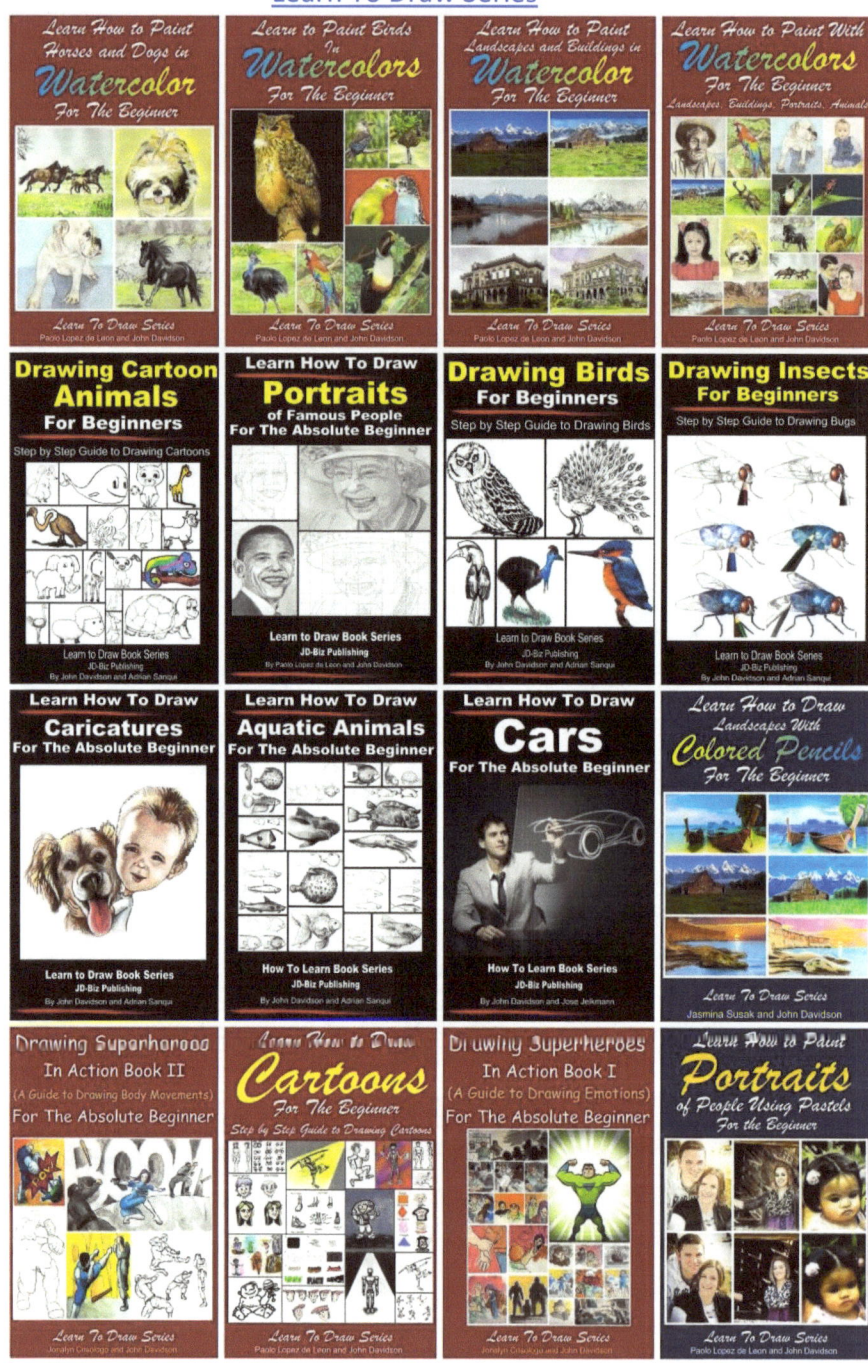

How to Build and Plan Books

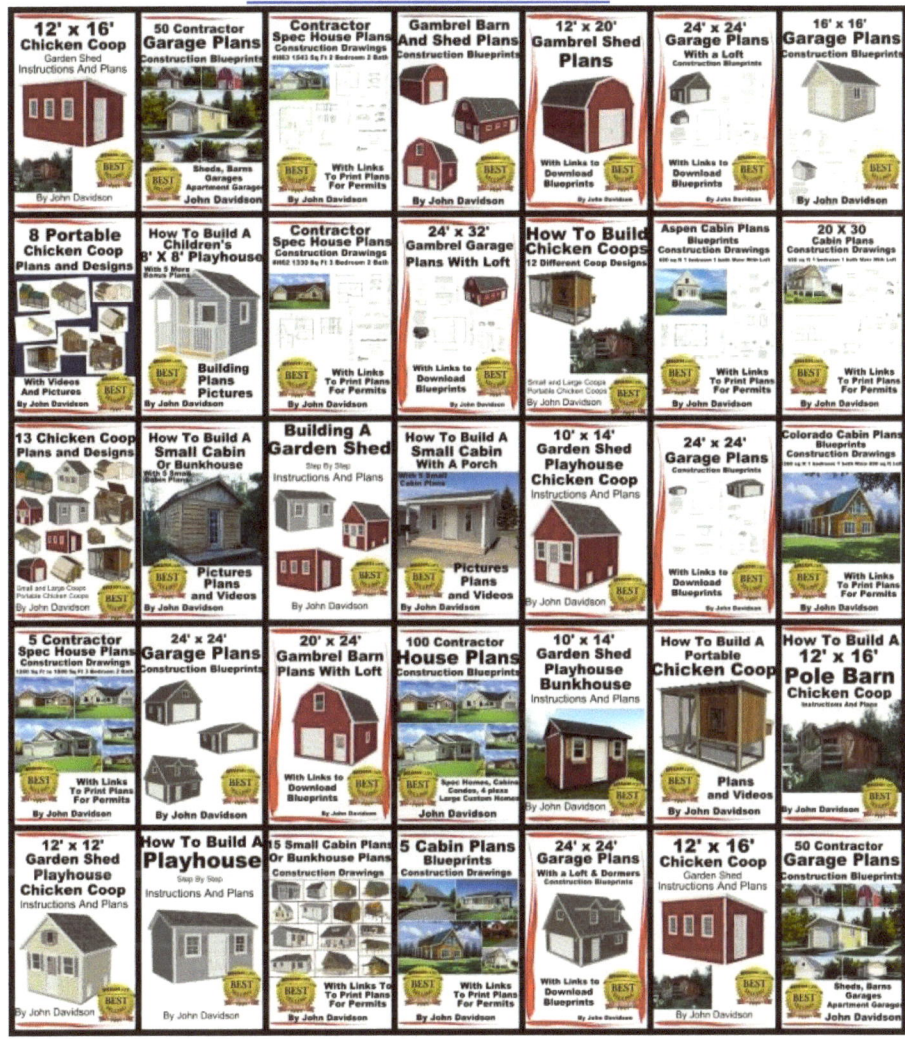

Entrepreneur Book Series

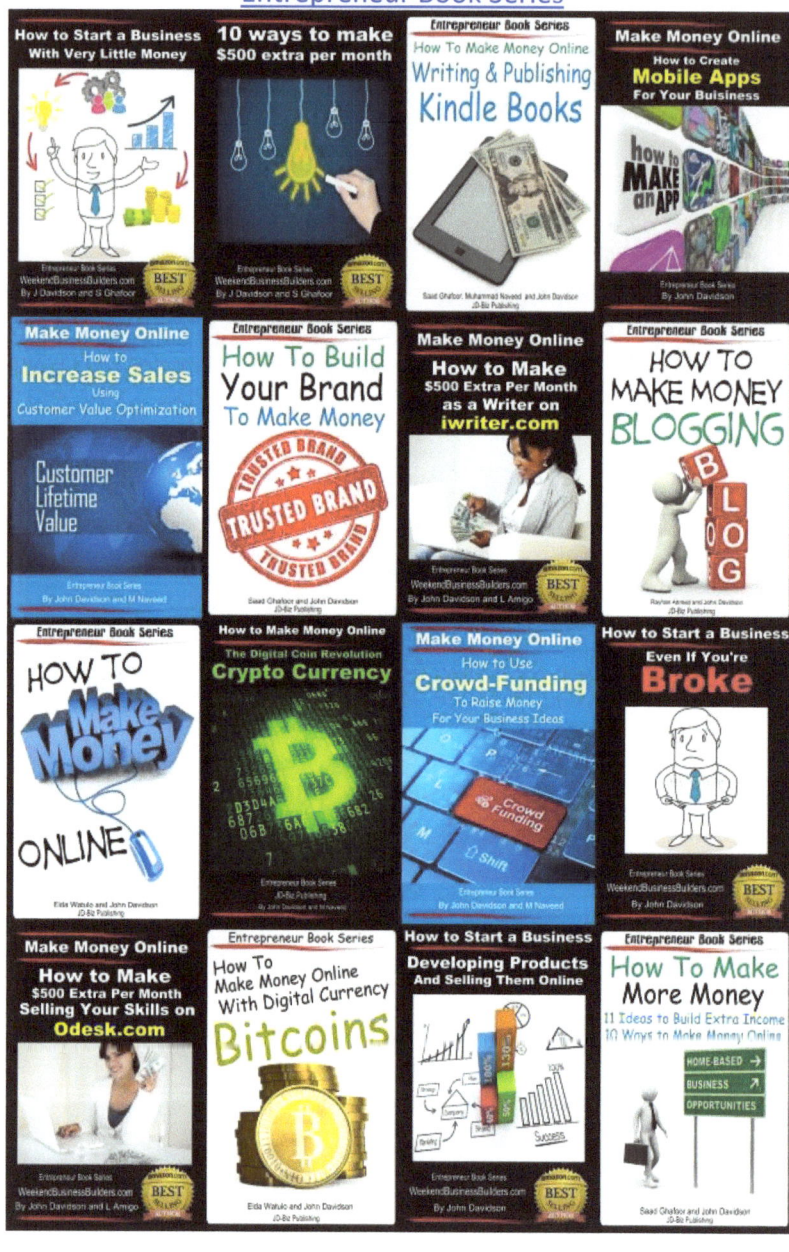

Our books are available at

1. Amazon.com
2. Barnes and Noble
3. Itunes
4. Kobo
5. Smashwords
6. Google Play Books

Download Free Books!
http://MendonCottageBooks.com

Publisher

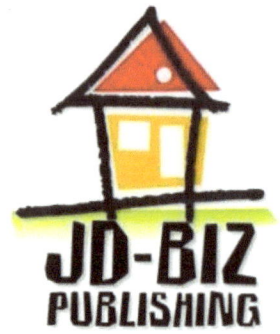

JD-Biz Corp

P O Box 374

Mendon, Utah 84325

http://www.jd-biz.com/

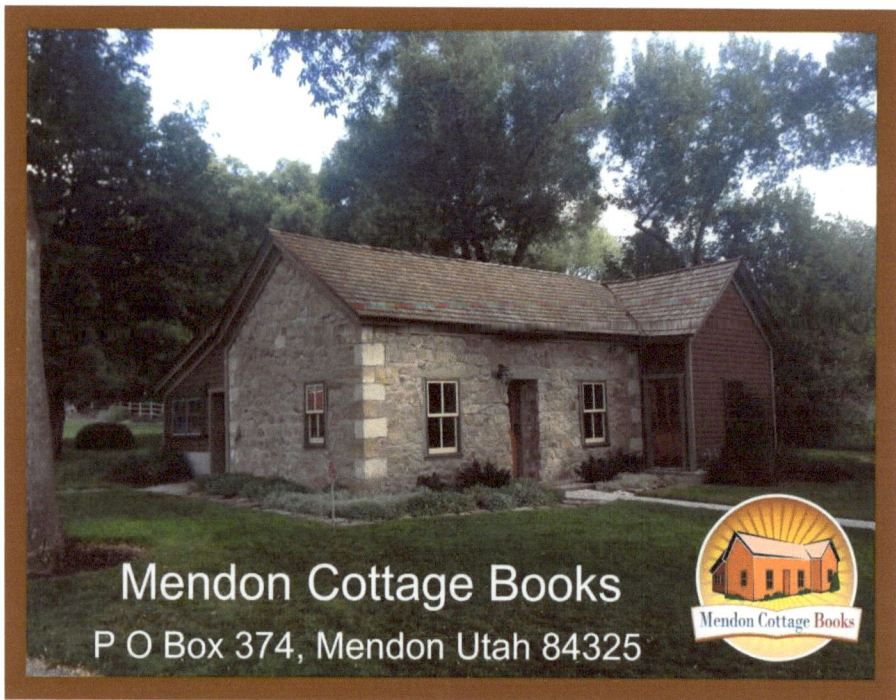

Mendon Cottage Books
P O Box 374, Mendon Utah 84325